Nutrition For A Vibrant Life

Enhance Energy Levels, Improve Mental Clarity, Reduce Risk of Chronic Diseases, and Optimize Your Long-term Health

Prem Sagar Sunchu

Your Free Gift !!

As a token of my thanks for taking out time to read my book, I would like to offer you a **Free-Gift**:

Click the Below Link and Download your **Free eBook PDF**.

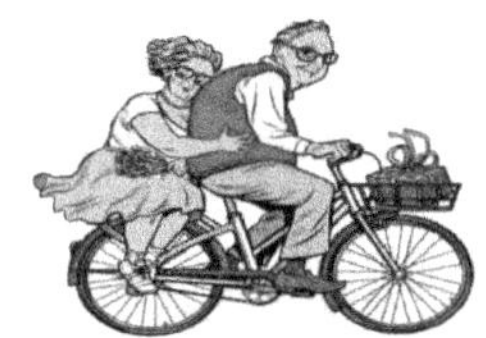

**Don't wait to be rich
to be happy
Happiness is free.**

"The Joyful Tapestry: A Global Mission for Happiness"

Or **Scan the QR Code** Below:

About The Author

Prem Sagar Sunchu, the Accomplished Author of "Nutrition for a Vibrant Life"

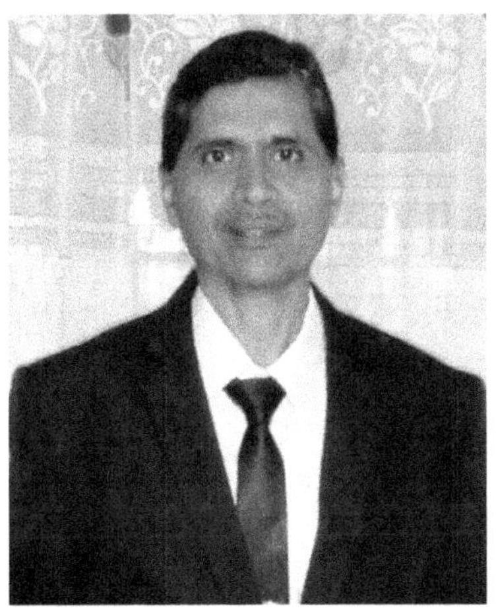

M eet Mr. Prem Sagar, an ordinary soul born in the vibrant city of Secunderabad, India, where the tapestry of life weaves stories of resilience and dreams. His journey is a testament to the power of perpetual learning, where every encounter is a lesson, and every moment holds the potential for growth.

A man of many dimensions, Mr. Sagar embodies the qualities of a perpetual student, a dedicated listener, and a dreamer who gazes at the stars but keeps his feet firmly grounded. His aspirations soar high, and his relentless pursuit of them is fueled by a genuine desire to make a positive impact on those around him.

Having served as a Chief Manager in the prestigious State Bank of India, Mr. Sagar brings a wealth of experience from the world of banking. However, for him, retirement isn't a conclusion but a commencement—a reminder that life's true journey begins when one can reflect on the wisdom gained from the first innings.

In Mr. Sagar's view, retirement is not a retreat but a stepping stone to a realm of infinite possibilities. It's an opportunity to surpass the ordinary, where the canvas of life awaits new brushstrokes of creativity and purpose. For him, the "be good and do good policy" isn't just a mantra; it's a guiding principle that shapes his approach to life.

As he embraces the second innings, Mr. Sagar encourages others to view retirement not as a winding down but as a springboard to new endeavors. It's a time when accumulated wisdom meets fresh energy, and the monotony of routine gives way to the vibrancy of creativity. His belief is clear: retirement is not just a number; it's a chapter where the richness of experience meets the possibilities in abundance.

In the world of Mr. Prem Sagar, retirement is not a period of rest but a canvas waiting to be painted with the colors of newfound wisdom, creativity, and a different outlook on life.

Prem Sagar Sunchu
M.Com, LLM, Certified Independent Director (IICA) GOI

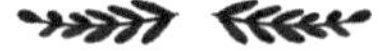

Acknowledgements

In profound gratitude, I extend heartfelt appreciation to my amazing parents. To my caring and resilient mother, **Smt. S.L. Lakshmi**, who gracefully navigated the challenges of my father's service transfers, made countless sacrifices to bind our family together. My father, **Shri S.R. Lakshman Rao**, stands as my enduring role model—his post-retirement vibrancy, marked by a dedicated hobby of reading and writing, serves as the very foundation that propels me into the realm of authorship.

A debt of gratitude is owed to my beautiful wife, **Smt. S.P. Padma Sree** is a constant source of inspiration, unwavering strength, and invaluable guidance. Balancing family responsibilities and the intricate path of an author, her presence has been the foundation of my journey.

To my handsome sons, **S.P. Gautam Sagar**, **S.P. Prayag Sagar**, and **S.P. Akshaj Sagar**, whose unwavering support and responsibility bear testament to the great strength they provide. Their motivation fuels my endeavors across all the diverse traits I undertake.

I owe thanks to **Mr. Som Bathla**, an **Amazon #1 Bestselling** author, for his mentorship, motivation, and guidance in the realms of **Writing, Self-Publishing, and Launching Books**. His support has been instrumental in initiating my journey as an Authorpreneur.

My Sincere thanks to **Mr. Sooraj Achar**, who is also an Amazon Bestselling Author, for his **Professional Editing,** Formatting, and Publishing support.

In acknowledging these pillars of support, I am reminded that the tapestry of my life and authorial pursuit is woven with threads of love, sacrifice, and inspiration. With profound thanks to my family, who stand as my bedrock of strength and motivation.

To the guiding stars of my universe—my Parents, Grandparents, Parents-in-law, Brothers, Sisters, the cherished members of our extended Family and Friends. Their unwavering support and boundless encouragement have been the driving force behind my Author Journey.

In the tapestry of my life, each of them has woven threads of inspiration and resilience, transforming mere words into stories and dreams into realities. Their confidence in me has been a constant source of strength, propelling me forward through the path of this journey.

With heartfelt gratitude, I dedicate the pages of my work to the pillars of love and encouragement that they are, recognizing that every word I pen is a tribute to the collective spirit of our family. May this dedication reflect the depth of my appreciation for the profound impact they have had on my creative journey.

"Nutrition for a Vibrant Life" is my second book in the series of five books-**"Holistic Well-being: A Journey to Balance"**

5.2 The Mediterranean Diet: A Blueprint for Longevity

5.3 Superfoods for Longevity and Disease Prevention

5.4 Incorporating Antioxidants for Cellular Health

5.5 The Role of Phytonutrients in Promoting Longevity

6. Practical Tips for Vibrant Eating   84

6.1 Meal Planning Strategies for Nutritious Eating

6.2 Smart Grocery Shopping: Reading Labels and Making Healthy Choices

6.3 Tips for Eating Out: Making Healthier Choices at Restaurants

6.4 Healthy Cooking Techniques: Grilling, Steaming, Roasting, and More

6.5 Building Balanced Meals: Sample Meal Ideas and Recipes

May I Ask You For A Small Favor?   101

Disclaimer   103

Introduction

Introduction: Unlocking the Path to Vibrant Living

In an era marked by an abundance of dietary information and choices, navigating the realm of nutrition can often feel like traversing a labyrinth without a map. Yet, at the heart of this complexity lies a simple truth: the food we eat holds the key to our health, vitality, and longevity.

This book, "Nourish," serves as your guiding light through this labyrinth, offering a comprehensive exploration of nutrition's fundamental principles and practical applications. Within its pages, you will embark on a journey of discovery, uncovering the profound impact of nutrition on every aspect of your life.

Chapter 1: Understanding Nutrition Basics

Our journey begins with a foundational understanding of nutrition basics. Here, we delve into the essential nutrients that fuel our bodies, unravel the mysteries of macronutrients and micronutrients, and explore the significance of balanced eating patterns. By grasping these fundamentals, you will lay the groundwork for informed dietary choices and optimal health.

Chapter 2: The Power of Whole Foods

Whole foods, untouched by processing and refinement, emerge as the unsung heroes of our diet. In this chapter, we celebrate the remarkable benefits of whole foods, from their abundance of essential nutrients to their potent disease-fighting properties. Through inspiring stories and compelling evidence, you will gain a newfound appreciation for the nourishing potential of nature's bounty.

Chapter 3: Nutrition and Energy Balance

Energy balance lies at the core of weight management and overall health. Here, we unravel the intricate interplay between calories consumed and calories expended, shedding light on the factors that influence our body weight and composition. Armed with this knowledge, you will learn to achieve and maintain a harmonious balance between energy intake and expenditure.

Chapter 4: Nutrition for Mental Well-being

The connection between nutrition and mental health is a burgeoning field of research, with profound implications for our emotional well-being. In this chapter, we explore the intimate relationship between diet and mental health, uncovering the nutrients that support cognitive function and mood regulation. By nurturing your brain with the right foods, you can cultivate resilience and vitality from within.

Chapter 5: Eating for Longevity

Longevity is not merely the absence of disease but the presence of energy and vitality. Here, we delve into the dietary strategies that promote longevity, from embracing anti-inflammatory foods to practicing mindful eating habits. By adopting a longevity-focused approach to nutrition, you can enrich your years and savor the gift of a vibrant life.

Chapter 6: Practical Tips for Vibrant Eating

Armed with knowledge and inspiration, we conclude our journey with practical tips for vibrant eating in the modern world. From navigating the grocery aisles to mastering the art of meal planning, you will discover actionable strategies for incorporating nutritious foods into your daily life. By making simple yet impactful changes, you can embark on a lifelong journey towards optimal health and vitality.

As you embark on this transformative journey through the pages of "Nourish," may you find wisdom, inspiration, and empowerment to nourish your body, mind, and soul. Together, let us unlock the extraordinary potential of nutrition and embrace the abundant blessings of vibrant living.

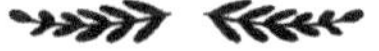

Understanding Nutrition Basics

*"Nutrition basics are the foundation upon which
we build our health, providing the blueprint for
vitality and longevity."*

1.1 Introduction to Macronutrients (Carbohydrates, Proteins, Fats)

Macronutrients, including carbohydrates, proteins, and fats, are the foundational components of our diet, providing the energy and substrates necessary for a myriad of physiological functions and maintaining homeostasis. Carbohydrates, composed of carbon, hydrogen, and oxygen atoms, are the primary source of energy for the body, with their complexity ranging from simple sugars to complex forms associated with fiber and starches.

- The intake of simple carbohydrates, or sugars, has been linked to decreased global cognition, while complex carbohydrates have been associated with improved memory and successful brain aging.

- Proteins, made up of amino acids linked by peptide bonds, not only serve as an energy source but are also crucial for tissue growth, repair, and cell signalling.

- They have been shown to enhance executive function and working memory, particularly under conditions of high cognitive demand.

- Fats, also composed of carbon, hydrogen, and oxygen, but with a lower proportion of oxygen, are essential for the structure of cells and the production of hormones.

- The type of fat consumed can have varying effects on health, with saturated fatty acids being linked to decreased memory and learning, while omega-3 fatty acids have a positive correlation with memory scores.

- The metabolism of these macronutrients is vital for normal organ function, thermoregulation, and physical activity.

- While macronutrients are primarily recognized for their role in providing energy, they are also substrates for metabolic pathways that are important for growth, development, and regulatory processes such as inflammation and immune reactions.

- The balance of macronutrient intake is critical, as it ensures that all of the body's nutritional requirements are met, and this balance can vary based on individual factors such as age, gender, weight, activity level, and general health status.

- A healthy diet that includes a variety of natural sources of fats, along with adequate proteins and carbohydrates, supports not only physical health but also cognitive function and brain integrity.

- Understanding the impact of macronutrient intake on both the body and the brain is key to developing nutritional recommendations that promote mental health and healthy aging.

1.2 Exploring Micronutrients (Vitamins and Minerals)

Introduction

Micronutrients, encompassing vitamins and minerals, are critical for numerous biological functions including growth, immune response, cognitive functions, and the regulation of gene expression. Despite their importance, there is a gap in understanding how these nutrients affect cognitive functioning and mental health.

Key Insights from Research Papers

- Micronutrients may significantly improve verbal cognitive abilities such as learning, flexibility, fluency, and inhibition in adults with ADHD and severe mood dysregulation, suggesting a link between nutrient intake and psychiatric functioning.

- Safe addition of micronutrients to foods can help address low micronutrient intakes in populations, with different safety levels established for various vitamins and minerals based on recommended daily intakes and tolerable upper intake levels.

- Comprehensive knowledge about micronutrients,

including their metabolic functions and the development of micronutrient-rich food products, is essential for maintaining health and preventing deficiencies.

Conclusion

The collective research underscores the potential of micronutrients to enhance cognitive and psychiatric functioning, particularly in individuals with specific mental health conditions. Additionally, the safe fortification of foods with micronutrients emerges as a viable strategy to combat deficiencies in the general population. Understanding the metabolic roles of these nutrients and incorporating them into a balanced diet is crucial for overall health maintenance.

1.3 The Role of Fiber in Digestive Health

Introduction

Dietary fiber plays a crucial role in maintaining digestive health through its diverse effects on the gastrointestinal system. It is a complex array of indigestible carbohydrates that influence gut motility, microbial diversity, immune responses, and systemic health.

Key Insights

- Dietary fibers, including complex carbohydrates and hydrocolloids, can slow upper gastrointestinal transit times, potentially affecting satiety and nutrient absorption, and serve as an energy source for gut microflora, impacting their diversity and toxicity.

- In children, specific fibers like partially hydrolyzed guar gum, glucomannan, and bran show beneficial effects on digestive health, but more research is needed, especially regarding whole-grain sources.

- Different physicochemical properties of dietary fibers, such as solubility, viscosity, and fermentability, are crucial for their functionality in the gut, affecting digestion, transit time, stool formation, and microbial composition, with implications for managing gastrointestinal disorders.

- Dietary fibers, including oligosaccharides, act as prebiotics, stimulating beneficial gut bacteria like Bifidobacterium and producing health-promoting metabolites like short-chain fatty acids.

- Beyond traditional benefits, dietary fibers may also play a role in immunomodulation, potentially aiding in infection prevention and improving mood and memory.

- In dogs and cats, dietary fiber is essential for gastrointestinal health, influencing appetite, digestion, and acting as a fermentable energy source for gut microbes, with systemic effects.

- The interaction of dietary fibers with gut microbes is pivotal for host physiology and health, with fiber-rich diets shaping microbial ecology and promoting beneficial metabolite production.

- The physiological effects of dietary fiber are closely linked to its behavior during digestion, including modulation of nutrient bioavailability, interaction with other food components, and fermentation in the large intestine.

- Increasing dietary fiber intake can affect the absorption of fats, nitrogen, energy, and minerals, with potential nutritional implications, including the impairment of calcium, zinc, and iron absorption.

- The physiological role of dietary fiber encompasses altering gut transit time, morphology, and flora, glucose tolerance, serum lipid levels, colon cancer risk, and mineral availability, with varying effects depending on the type of fiber.

Conclusion

Dietary fiber is integral to digestive health, with its benefits extending to satiety, gut microflora diversity, immune function, and the prevention of various diseases. The type and source of fiber, along with its physicochemical properties, determine its specific effects on the gastrointestinal system. While certain fibers have been shown to be beneficial, the optimal types and amounts for health and disease management remain areas for further research. Additionally, the impact of fiber on nutrient absorption highlights the need for a balanced approach when increasing fiber intake.

1.4 Importance of Hydration and Water Balance

Introduction

Hydration and water balance are critical for maintaining human health, as water plays a fundamental role in various physiological processes. Understanding the importance of hydration involves examining the body's water requirements, the consequences of dehydration, and the factors influencing water balance.

Key Insights on Hydration and Water Balance

- Water is essential for numerous bodily functions, including acting as a building material, solvent, carrier for nutrients and waste, thermoregulation, and lubrication; precise regulation of water balance is crucial for health, with recommendations for a sedentary adult to drink 1.5 liters per day.

- The body's water content is significant, making up a large percentage of nonfat weight and total weight, with water being critical for metabolic reactions, nutrient transport, and maintaining blood volume and fluid balance.

- Hydration status can be influenced by internal factors like a lack of thirst sensation or external factors such as medication use, with drugs and excipients potentially affecting water balance through various mechanisms.

- Adequate hydration is associated with reduced risks of certain diseases, and proper timing of water intake may contribute to weight management; however, the specific benefits of hydration on various aspects of health require further research.

- Various techniques exist to assess hydration status, including isotope dilution, bioelectrical impedance, and urinary markers, which are important for ensuring accurate evaluation of body fluid compartments.

- During the COVID-19 pandemic, a study found that young adults in Turkey maintained a positive net water balance, highlighting the importance of hydration, especially during infectious diseases.

- Optimal hydration levels are crucial for wound healing, with a moist environment supporting the healing process and the need for dressings that manage wound fluid effectively.

- Maintaining proper hydration status is vital for cognitive function and overall health, with various biomarkers available to evaluate hydration status and the need for health education on adequate water intake.

- Thirst may not always be a reliable indicator for hydration needs in certain populations, such as infants, athletes, the ill, and the elderly, and the consumption of certain beverages can influence overall hydration.

- Healthy older adults can maintain water balance and hydration status comparable to younger adults, with no significant differences in water input, output, or net balance, although fat-free mass hydration appears to be higher in older individuals.

Conclusion

Maintaining proper hydration is essential for a wide range of bodily functions and can influence health outcomes.

While the body has mechanisms to regulate water balance, certain populations may require more careful monitoring and scheduled water intake. Both the quantity and timing of water consumption can have implications for disease prevention and weight management. Assessment techniques are available to monitor hydration status, which is particularly important for vulnerable groups and in the context of health conditions such as infectious diseases and wound healing. Overall, hydration remains a key component of health across all age groups.

1.5 Understanding Nutrient Density and its Significance

Introduction

Nutrient density is a concept that evaluates the nutritional value of foods, diets, or meals in relation to their energy content. It is particularly important in ensuring that dietary regimens meet the specific nutritional needs of individuals or target groups, especially when energy intake is low.

Key Insights

- Nutrient density is crucial for diets with low energy intake to cover the requirements of certain nutrients, such as iron, which is absorbed based on its bioavailability and the iron status of individuals.

- Dietetic regimens require higher nutrient density compared to normal diets, especially for nutrients like protein, calcium, iron, vitamin B1, and vitamin C, to meet specific energy and nutrient demands.

- The Nutrient Rich Foods (NRF) index defines nutrient density formally, ranking foods based on their nutritional value using a metric that includes nutrients to encourage and limit, thus guiding healthier food choices.

- In broiler chickens, increasing dietary nutrient density, while maintaining essential nutrients in proportion to energy, improves feed conversion and affects body weight and carcass quality, indicating the broader implications of nutrient density in animal nutrition.

Conclusion

Nutrient density is a key factor in assessing the nutritional quality of foods and diets, ensuring that nutritional needs are met even when energy intake is restricted.

It is particularly significant in specialized diets that require higher concentrations of certain nutrients. The NRF index provides a validated method to quantify and rank the nutrient density of foods, aiding in the selection of nutrient-rich options.

Additionally, the concept of nutrient density extends to animal nutrition, where it influences growth performance and carcass characteristics.

13

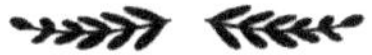

The Power of Whole Foods

2.1 Benefits of Whole Grains and Their Varieties

"Whole grains are not just food; they are a foundation for a healthy lifestyle, offering a wealth of nutrients and health benefits that nourish both body and mind." - Unknown

Introduction:

Whole grains stand as nutritional powerhouses, offering an array of health benefits that make them indispensable in a balanced diet. From their high fiber content to their rich vitamin and mineral profiles, whole grains play a crucial role in promoting overall health and well-being.

Understanding the significance of whole grains and their varieties is essential for making informed dietary choices that support long-term health.

Key Insights:

1. Fiber-Rich Nutrition: Whole grains are renowned for their high fiber content, which supports digestive health, aids in weight management, and regulates blood sugar levels. The combination of soluble and insoluble fiber in whole grains contributes to feelings of fullness, promotes regular bowel movements, and helps prevent constipation and other digestive issues.

2. Heart Health Benefits: Research consistently shows that diets rich in whole grains are associated with a reduced risk of heart disease. Whole grains help lower cholesterol levels, reduce blood pressure, and decrease inflammation—all factors that contribute to improved cardiovascular health. The fiber, antioxidants, and other bioactive compounds found in whole grains work synergistically to support heart health and reduce the risk of heart disease.

3. Weight Management Support: Whole grains can be valuable allies in weight management efforts due to their satiating effect and slow digestion rate. By promoting feelings of fullness and preventing rapid spikes in blood sugar levels, whole grains help individuals control appetite and reduce overall calorie intake.

Incorporating whole grains into meals can support weight loss goals and contribute to a balanced diet.

4. Diabetes Prevention and Management: Consuming whole grains is linked to a lower risk of type 2 diabetes and better blood sugar control in individuals with diabetes. The fiber and complex carbohydrates in whole grains help regulate blood sugar levels, improve insulin sensitivity, and reduce the risk of insulin resistance—a hallmark of type 2 diabetes. Including whole grains in the diet can play a significant role in diabetes prevention and management.

5. Nutrient Density: Whole grains are packed with essential nutrients, including vitamins, minerals, and antioxidants. They provide key nutrients such as B vitamins (thiamin, riboflavin, niacin, and folate), magnesium, iron, zinc, and selenium, which are vital for energy metabolism, immune function, and overall health. By incorporating a variety of whole grains into the diet, individuals can ensure they receive a diverse array of nutrients essential for optimal health.

Conclusion:

Incorporating whole grains and their varieties into the diet offers a multitude of health benefits, ranging from improved digestive health and heart health to weight management and diabetes prevention. The fiber, vitamins, minerals, and antioxidants found in whole grains support overall health and well-being, making them an essential component of a balanced diet. By prioritizing whole grains over refined grains and incorporating a diverse range of whole grain options into meals, individuals can optimize their nutrient intake and promote long-term health and vitality.

Resources:

1. Harvard T.H. Chan School of Public Health. "The Nutrition Source: Whole Grains." (https://www.hsph.harvard.edu/nutritionsource/what-should-you-eat/whole-grains/)

2. Whole Grains Council. "Health Benefits of Whole Grains." (https://wholegrainscouncil.org/health-benefits-of-whole-grains)

3. Mayo Clinic. "Whole grains: Hearty options for a healthy diet." (https://www.mayoclinic.org/healthy-lifestyle/nutrition-and-healthy-eating/in-depth/whole-grains/art-20047826)

2.2 Incorporating Fresh Fruits and Vegetables for Optimal Health

"Let food be thy medicine and medicine be thy food."
- Hippocrates

Introduction:

Incorporating fresh fruits and vegetables into one's diet is essential for achieving optimal health and vitality. Fruits and vegetables are rich sources of vitamins, minerals, fiber, and antioxidants, all of which play critical roles in supporting various bodily functions and preventing chronic diseases. Understanding the importance of incorporating these nutrient-dense foods and exploring strategies to increase their consumption is paramount for promoting overall well-being.

Key Insights:

1. Nutrient-Rich Powerhouses: Fresh fruits and vegetables are nutritional powerhouses, providing essential vitamins, minerals, and phytonutrients necessary for maintaining health and preventing disease. They are particularly rich in vitamin C, vitamin A, potassium, folate, and dietary fiber, all of which contribute to overall well-being.

2. Disease Prevention: A diet rich in fruits and vegetables has been associated with a reduced risk of chronic diseases, including heart disease, stroke, type 2 diabetes, and certain types of cancer. The diverse array of antioxidants found in fruits and vegetables helps combat oxidative stress and inflammation, which are underlying factors in the development of chronic diseases.

3. Weight Management: Fruits and vegetables are low in calories and high in fiber, making them valuable tools for weight management. Their high water content adds volume to meals, helping individuals feel full and satisfied with fewer calories. Incorporating a variety of fruits and vegetables into meals and snacks can support weight loss efforts and promote a healthy body weight.

4. Digestive Health: The fiber content in fruits and vegetables supports digestive health by promoting regular bowel movements and preventing constipation. Fiber also acts as a prebiotic, nourishing beneficial bacteria in the gut and promoting a healthy gut microbiome. A healthy gut microbiome is essential for optimal digestion, nutrient absorption, and immune function.

5. Mental Well-being: Emerging research suggests a link between fruit and vegetable consumption and mental well-being. Diets rich in fruits and vegetables have been associated with a lower risk of depression and anxiety, as well as improved cognitive function and overall mood. The nutrients and antioxidants found in fruits and vegetables support brain health and may contribute to better mental health outcomes.

Conclusion:

Incorporating fresh fruits and vegetables into the diet is crucial for achieving optimal health and preventing chronic diseases.

These nutrient-dense foods provide a wide range of vitamins, minerals, fiber, and antioxidants that support various bodily functions and promote overall well-being. By prioritizing the consumption of fruits and vegetables and diversifying the types and colors consumed, individuals can optimize their nutrient intake and enjoy the numerous health benefits associated with these plant-based foods.

Resources:

1. Harvard T.H. Chan School of Public Health. "The Nutrition Source - Vegetables and Fruits." (https://www.hsph.harvard.edu/nutritionsource/what-should-you-eat/vegetables-and-fruits/)

2. Centers for Disease Control and Prevention (CDC). "Fruits and Vegetables." (https://www.cdc.gov/nutrition/fruits/index.html)

3. American Heart Association. "Vegetables and Fruits." (https://www.heart.org/en/healthy-living/healthy-eating/add-color/vegetables-and-fruits)

2.3 The Importance of Lean Proteins and Plant-Based Alternatives

"The food you eat can be either the safest and most powerful form of medicine or the slowest form of poison." - Ann Wigmore

Introduction:

The importance of incorporating lean proteins and plant-based alternatives into one's diet cannot be overstated in the pursuit of optimal health and nutrition. Proteins are essential macronutrients necessary for various bodily functions, including muscle building, repair, and hormone synthesis. While lean animal proteins have traditionally been emphasized, plant-based alternatives offer numerous health benefits and cater to diverse dietary preferences and ethical considerations. Understanding the significance of both lean proteins and plant-based options is crucial for maintaining a balanced and sustainable diet.

Key Insights:

1. Muscle Health and Maintenance: Proteins, regardless of their source, are vital for maintaining muscle health and supporting

overall physical function. They provide essential amino acids necessary for muscle protein synthesis, repair, and growth. Incorporating lean protein sources like poultry, fish, tofu, legumes, and low-fat dairy into meals helps meet daily protein requirements, supporting muscle health, especially in physically active individuals and those engaged in resistance training.

2. Weight Management: Protein plays a crucial role in weight management by promoting satiety, regulating appetite, and preserving lean body mass. Lean protein sources, such as poultry, fish, tofu, legumes, and low-fat dairy, help individuals feel full and satisfied, reducing the likelihood of overeating and supporting weight loss or weight maintenance efforts. Plant-based protein alternatives like beans, lentils, quinoa, and tempeh offer similar satiety and nutritional benefits while being lower in saturated fat and cholesterol.

3. Heart Health: Choosing lean protein sources over fatty or processed meats can significantly benefit heart health. Lean proteins, particularly those from poultry, fish, and plant-based sources, are lower in saturated fat and cholesterol, which are risk factors for heart disease. Plant-based protein alternatives often contain heart-healthy nutrients such as fiber, antioxidants, and unsaturated fats, further supporting cardiovascular health and reducing the risk of heart disease.

4. Environmental Sustainability: Plant-based protein alternatives are gaining popularity not only for their health

benefits but also for their environmental sustainability. Compared to animal agriculture, plant-based protein production typically requires fewer resources, produces fewer greenhouse gas emissions, and has a lower environmental impact. Opting for plant-based protein options over animal products can help reduce the ecological footprint of one's diet and contribute to a more sustainable food system.

5. Diverse Nutritional Benefits: Plant-based protein alternatives offer a diverse array of nutritional benefits beyond protein content. They are rich sources of fiber, vitamins, minerals, and phytonutrients, which are essential for overall health and disease prevention. By incorporating a variety of plant-based protein sources into their diets, individuals can ensure they receive a wide range of nutrients while reducing their reliance on animal products.

Conclusion:

Incorporating both lean proteins and plant-based alternatives into one's diet is crucial for achieving a balanced and nutritious eating pattern. These protein sources offer unique advantages for health, sustainability, and dietary diversity. Whether sourced from lean animal proteins or plant-based options, protein remains essential for muscle health, weight management, heart health, and overall well-being. By embracing a variety of lean proteins and plant-based alternatives in their meals, individuals can optimize their nutrient intake, align with health goals, and contribute to a more sustainable food ecosystem. Flexibility and diversity in protein choices empower individuals to tailor their diets to meet nutritional needs, preferences, and ethical considerations, ultimately fostering long-term health and vitality.

Resources:

1. Harvard T.H. Chan School of Public Health. "Protein." (https://www.hsph.harvard.edu/nutritionsource/what-should-you-eat/protein/)

2. Academy of Nutrition and Dietetics. "Vegetarian Nutrition." (https://www.eatright.org/food/nutrition/vegetarian-and-special-diets/vegetarian-nutrition)

3. American Heart Association. "Meat, Poultry, and Fish: Picking Healthy Proteins."

2.4 Nuts, Seeds, and Healthy Fats: Their Role in a Balanced Diet

"Those who think they have no time for healthy eating will sooner or later have to find time for illness." - Edward Stanley

Introduction:

Nuts, seeds, and healthy fats play a pivotal role in a balanced diet, offering an array of essential nutrients and contributing to overall health and well-being. Despite their high calorie content, these foods are rich in heart-healthy fats, vitamins, minerals, and antioxidants, making them valuable components of a nutritious eating pattern. Understanding the role of nuts, seeds, and healthy fats in promoting health and exploring strategies to incorporate them into the diet is essential for optimizing nutrition and achieving long-term wellness.

Key Insights:

1. Heart Health Benefits: Nuts and seeds are rich sources of unsaturated fats, including monounsaturated and polyunsaturated fats, which have been associated with improved heart health. Regular consumption of nuts and seeds has been linked to lower cholesterol levels, reduced inflammation, and decreased risk of heart disease. Additionally, the omega-3 fatty acids found in certain nuts and seeds, such as walnuts and flaxseeds, offer further cardiovascular benefits, including decreased risk of arrhythmias and improved blood vessel function.

2. Nutrient Density: Nuts and seeds are nutrient-dense foods, packed with vitamins, minerals, and antioxidants. They provide

essential nutrients such as vitamin E, magnesium, potassium, and zinc, which support immune function, bone health, and overall well-being. Incorporating a variety of nuts and seeds into the diet ensures a diverse array of nutrients and phytonutrients, promoting optimal health and vitality.

3. Weight Management Support: Despite their relatively high calorie content, nuts, seeds, and healthy fats can aid in weight management when consumed in moderation. The combination of protein, fiber, and healthy fats in nuts and seeds helps promote satiety, preventing overeating and supporting weight loss efforts. Studies have shown that including nuts and seeds in the diet can lead to better weight management outcomes and reduced risk of obesity.

4. Diabetes Management: Nuts, seeds, and healthy fats may play a beneficial role in diabetes management. Their low glycemic index and high fiber content help regulate blood sugar levels, improve insulin sensitivity, and reduce the risk of type 2 diabetes. Incorporating nuts and seeds into meals and snacks can contribute to better glycemic control and overall diabetes management.

5. Brain Health: The nutrients and antioxidants found in nuts, seeds, and healthy fats support brain health and cognitive function. Omega-3 fatty acids, in particular, are essential for brain development and function, and regular consumption of

nuts and seeds may help reduce the risk of age-related cognitive decline and improve memory and learning.

Conclusion:

Nuts, seeds, and healthy fats are valuable components of a balanced diet, offering numerous health benefits and contributing to overall well-being. Their rich nutrient profiles, including heart-healthy fats, vitamins, minerals, and antioxidants, make them essential for promoting heart health, supporting weight management, and reducing the risk of chronic diseases such as heart disease, diabetes, and obesity. By incorporating a variety of nuts, seeds, and healthy fats into meals and snacks, individuals can optimize their nutrient intake, enhance satiety, and improve overall health and vitality.

Resources:

1. Harvard T.H. Chan School of Public Health. "Nuts for the Heart: An Overview of the Research." (https://www.hsph.harvard.edu/nutritionsource/nuts-for-the-heart/)

2. American Heart Association.
"Nuts, Seeds and Heart Health." (https://www.heart.org/en/healthy-living/healthy-eating/eat-smart/fats/nuts-and-seeds)

3. Mayo Clinic. "Nuts and your heart: Eating nuts for heart health."

2.5 Exploring the Benefits of Herbs, Spices, and Seasonings

"Herbs and spices are not just condiments; they are nature's pharmacy, offering a treasure trove of health benefits in every sprinkle and dash." - Unknown

Introduction:

Herbs, spices, and seasonings have been integral to culinary traditions worldwide for centuries, not only for their ability to enhance flavor but also for their potential health benefits. Beyond adding taste and aroma to dishes, these plant-based ingredients are rich sources of phytochemicals, antioxidants, and other bioactive compounds that contribute to overall well-being. Exploring the benefits of herbs, spices, and seasonings sheds light on their potential roles in promoting health and vitality.

Key Insights:

1. Antioxidant Properties: Many herbs, spices, and seasonings boast potent antioxidant properties due to their high content of polyphenols, flavonoids, and other antioxidants. These compounds help neutralize harmful free radicals in the body, reducing oxidative stress and inflammation, and lowering the risk of chronic diseases such as heart disease, cancer, and neurodegenerative disorders.

2. Anti-inflammatory Effects: Certain herbs and spices exhibit anti-inflammatory properties, which can help alleviate inflammation and associated symptoms in conditions like arthritis, asthma, and inflammatory bowel diseases. For example, turmeric contains curcumin, a compound renowned for its anti-inflammatory and pain-relieving effects.

3. Digestive Health: Many herbs and spices have been traditionally used to aid digestion and alleviate gastrointestinal discomfort. For instance, ginger and peppermint are known for their ability to ease nausea, bloating, and indigestion. Additionally, herbs like thyme, rosemary, and oregano contain compounds that may support digestive function and inhibit the growth of harmful bacteria in the gut.

4. Blood Sugar Regulation: Some herbs and spices have been shown to help regulate blood sugar levels and improve insulin sensitivity, making them beneficial for individuals with diabetes

or those at risk of developing the condition. Cinnamon, for example, has been found to lower blood glucose levels by enhancing insulin action and improving glucose metabolism.

5. Cognitive Function: Certain herbs and spices may have positive effects on cognitive function and brain health. For instance, research suggests that sage may improve memory and cognitive performance, while cinnamon and turmeric have been studied for their potential to protect against age-related cognitive decline and neurodegenerative diseases like Alzheimer's.

Conclusion:

Exploring the benefits of herbs, spices, and seasonings reveals their potential to enhance both the flavor and nutritional value of meals while promoting health and well-being. From their antioxidant and anti-inflammatory properties to their role in supporting digestive health, regulating blood sugar levels, and improving cognitive function, herbs and spices offer a wealth of health benefits. By incorporating a variety of herbs, spices, and seasonings into daily cooking and meal preparation, individuals can not only enjoy delicious and flavorful dishes but also harness the therapeutic potential of these plant-based ingredients to optimize health and vitality.

Resources:

1. National Center for Complementary and Integrative Health (NCCIH). "Herbs at a Glance." (https://www.nccih.nih.gov/health/herbsat-a-glance)

2. American Heart Association.
"How to Add Flavor Without Adding Sodium." (https://www.heart.org/en/healthy-living/healthy-eating/eat-smart/sodium/how-to-add-flavor-without-adding-sodium)

3. Academy of Nutrition and Dietetics. "Herbs and Spices." (https://www.eatright.org/food/vitamins-and-supplements/nutrient-rich-foods/herbs-and-spices)

Nutrition and Energy Balance

3.1 Understanding Caloric Needs and Energy Expenditure

"It's not just about eating less; it's about eating right."
- Unknown

Introduction:

Understanding caloric needs and energy expenditure is fundamental to maintaining a healthy weight and overall well-being. Calories are units of energy derived from the foods and beverages we consume, and our bodies require a certain number of calories to function optimally each day. However, individual caloric needs vary based on factors such as age, gender, weight, height, activity level, and metabolic rate. By gaining insight into caloric requirements and energy expenditure, individuals can make informed decisions about their diet and lifestyle to support their health goals.

Key Insights:

1. Basal Metabolic Rate (BMR): Basal metabolic rate refers to the number of calories the body needs to perform basic functions such as breathing, circulating blood, and maintaining body temperature while at rest. BMR accounts for the largest proportion of total energy expenditure, typically representing 60-70% of total daily energy expenditure.

2. Physical Activity Level: Physical activity, including exercise, work-related activities, and daily movement, significantly influences total energy expenditure. The more physically active a person is, the higher their caloric needs will be to fuel these activities. Individuals engaging in regular exercise or strenuous physical labor may require more calories to meet their energy demands.

3. Thermic Effect of Food (TEF): The thermic effect of food refers to the energy expenditure associated with digesting, absorbing, and metabolizing nutrients from food. Different macronutrients have varying thermic effects, with protein requiring more energy to digest compared to carbohydrates and fats. Including a balance of macronutrients in meals can

optimize the thermic effect of food and support overall energy expenditure.

4. Factors Affecting Caloric Needs: Several factors influence individual caloric needs and energy expenditure, including age, gender, body composition, genetics, hormonal fluctuations, and medical conditions. For example, younger individuals and those with higher lean muscle mass typically have higher caloric needs than older adults or individuals with lower muscle mass.

5. Balancing Energy Intake and Expenditure: Achieving energy balance—where energy intake equals energy expenditure—is essential for weight maintenance. Consuming more calories than the body expends leads to weight gain, while consuming fewer calories than expended results in weight loss. Understanding caloric needs and adjusting dietary intake and physical activity levels accordingly can help individuals achieve and maintain a healthy weight.

Conclusion:

Understanding caloric needs and energy expenditure is crucial for maintaining a healthy weight and supporting overall health and well-being. By recognizing the factors that influence caloric requirements, individuals can make informed decisions about their diet and lifestyle to achieve energy balance and meet their health goals. Balancing energy intake with expenditure through mindful eating, regular physical activity, and awareness of individual needs can promote optimal health and vitality in the long term.

Resources:

1. Centers for Disease Control and Prevention (CDC). "Balancing Calories." (https://www.cdc.gov/healthyweight/healthy_eating/calories.html)

2. Academy of Nutrition and Dietetics. "Understanding Calories." (https://www.eatright.org/health/weight-loss/calories/understanding-calories)

3. Mayo Clinic. "Counting Calories: Get Back to Weight-loss Basics."

3.2 Balanced Meals: Creating a Plate with Proper Proportions

"Every time you eat or drink, you are either feeding disease or fighting it." - Heather Morgan

Introduction:

Creating balanced meals with proper proportions is essential for promoting overall health and providing the body with the nutrients it needs to function optimally. A balanced plate incorporates a variety of food groups in appropriate proportions, including fruits, vegetables, lean proteins, whole grains, and healthy fats. Understanding how to create balanced meals ensures that individuals meet their nutritional needs, maintain energy levels, and support long-term well-being.

Key Insights:

1. The Plate Method: The plate method is a simple and effective tool for creating balanced meals. It involves dividing the plate into sections and filling each section with specific food groups:

- Half the plate should consist of fruits and vegetables, providing essential vitamins, minerals, and fiber.

- One-quarter of the plate should contain lean proteins, such as poultry, fish, tofu, legumes, or lean cuts of meat, to support muscle health and repair.

- The remaining quarter of the plate should include whole grains or starchy vegetables, such as brown rice, quinoa, whole wheat pasta, or sweet potatoes, for sustained energy and fiber.

- A small portion of healthy fats, such as olive oil, avocado, or nuts, can complement the meal and provide essential fatty acids and fat-soluble vitamins.

2. Nutrient Density: Balancing meals with a variety of nutrient-dense foods ensures that individuals receive a wide range of essential nutrients necessary for overall health and well-being. Nutrient-dense foods are those that provide a high amount of nutrients relative to their calorie content. Incorporating a colorful array of fruits and vegetables, lean proteins, whole grains, and healthy fats into meals maximizes nutrient intake and supports optimal health.

3. Portion Control: Proper portion control is key to creating balanced meals and preventing overeating. While the plate method provides a general guideline for portion sizes, individual calorie needs and activity levels should also be considered. Paying attention to hunger and fullness cues, eating mindfully, and practicing portion control can help individuals maintain a healthy weight and prevent weight gain.

4. Dietary Diversity: Including a variety of foods from different food groups ensures dietary diversity and provides a wide range of nutrients, flavors, and textures. Aim to incorporate different types of fruits, vegetables, proteins, grains, and fats into meals to promote overall health and enjoyment of food. Experimenting with new recipes, cuisines, and cooking techniques can help

increase dietary diversity and make meals more exciting and satisfying.

Conclusion:

Creating balanced meals with proper proportions is essential for supporting overall health, providing essential nutrients, and maintaining energy levels. The plate method offers a simple and practical approach to balancing meals, ensuring that individuals include a variety of fruits, vegetables, lean proteins, whole grains, and healthy fats in their diet. By paying attention to portion sizes, practicing portion control, and focusing on dietary diversity, individuals can optimize their nutrition, promote satiety, and support long-term well-being.

Resources:

1. MyPlate. "10 Tips: Build a Healthy Meal." (https://www.myplate.gov/eat-healthy/10-tips-build-healthy-m eal)

2. American Heart Association.
"Healthy Eating: Portion Control." (https://www.heart.org/en/healthy-living/healthy-eating/eat-s mart/nutrition-basics/portion-control)

3. Harvard T.H. Chan School of Public Health. "The Nutrition Source - Healthy Eating Plate."

3.3 The Impact of Sugars and Sweeteners on Energy Levels

"The energy you need comes from the choices you make." - Unknown

Introduction:

The impact of sugars and sweeteners on energy levels is a topic of significant interest due to their prevalence in the modern diet and their potential effects on health and well-being. While sugars provide a quick source of energy, excessive consumption can lead to energy crashes and long-term health consequences such as obesity and type 2 diabetes. On the other hand, artificial sweeteners are marketed as low-calorie alternatives but may have unintended effects on metabolism and energy regulation. Understanding the complex relationship between sugars, sweeteners, and energy levels is essential for making informed dietary choices and promoting overall health.

Key Insights:

1. Sugars and Blood Sugar Levels: Consuming foods and beverages high in sugars can cause rapid spikes in blood sugar levels, followed by subsequent crashes. These fluctuations in

blood sugar can lead to feelings of fatigue, irritability, and decreased energy levels. While sugars provide a quick source of energy, their rapid absorption can disrupt blood sugar regulation and contribute to metabolic dysregulation over time.

2. Effects of Added Sugars: Added sugars, such as sucrose and high-fructose corn syrup, are prevalent in processed foods and beverages and contribute significantly to daily caloric intake. Excessive consumption of added sugars has been linked to weight gain, obesity, insulin resistance, and an increased risk of type 2 diabetes. Limiting intake of foods and drinks high in added sugars can help stabilize energy levels and promote overall health.

3. Artificial Sweeteners and Metabolic Effects: Artificial sweeteners, such as aspartame, sucralose, and stevia, are widely used as low-calorie alternatives to sugar. While they provide sweetness without adding calories, research suggests that artificial sweeteners may have unintended effects on metabolism and energy regulation. Some studies have found associations between artificial sweetener consumption and increased appetite, altered gut microbiota, and metabolic dysregulation, although further research is needed to elucidate these effects fully.

4. Balancing Sweeteners in the Diet: Achieving a balance between sugars and sweeteners is crucial for maintaining stable energy levels and promoting overall health. While sugars provide

quick energy, they should be consumed in moderation and preferably in their natural form, such as fruits and vegetables, which also provide essential nutrients and fiber. Artificial sweeteners can be used sparingly as part of a balanced diet but should not replace whole, nutrient-dense foods.

Conclusion:

The impact of sugars and sweeteners on energy levels is complex, with both providing potential benefits and risks depending on consumption patterns and individual health status. While sugars offer quick energy, excessive intake can lead to energy crashes and metabolic disturbances. Artificial sweeteners may provide sweetness without calories but may have unintended effects on metabolism and appetite regulation. Achieving a balance between sugars and sweeteners by prioritizing whole, nutrient-dense foods and limiting consumption of added sugars and artificial sweeteners is essential for maintaining stable energy levels and promoting overall health.

Resources:

1. Centers for Disease Control and Prevention (CDC). "Added Sugars." (https://www.cdc.gov/nutrition/data-statistics/plain-water-the-healthier-choice.html)

2. Harvard T.H. Chan School of Public Health. "The Nutrition Source - Added Sugars." (https://www.hsph.harvard.edu/nutritionsource/healthy-drinks/sugary-drinks/)

3. American Heart Association. "Artificial Sweeteners."

3.4 Timing Meals and Snacks for Sustained Energy

"Eat breakfast like a king, lunch like a prince, and dinner like a pauper." - Adelle Davis

Introduction:

Timing meals and snacks appropriately throughout the day is crucial for sustaining energy levels, optimizing performance, and supporting overall health and well-being. By understanding the impact of meal timing on energy metabolism and blood sugar regulation, individuals can make informed choices about when to eat to maintain stable energy levels and promote optimal functioning of the body and mind.

Key Insights:

1. Balancing Blood Sugar Levels: Eating regular meals and snacks at consistent intervals helps stabilize blood sugar levels throughout the day, preventing energy dips and fluctuations. Consuming a combination of carbohydrates, proteins, and healthy fats at each meal can slow the absorption of sugars into the bloodstream, providing sustained energy over time.

2. Importance of Breakfast: Breakfast is often referred to as the most important meal of the day as it jumpstarts metabolism, replenishes energy stores after an overnight fast, and provides essential nutrients to fuel the body and brain. A balanced breakfast that includes protein, whole grains, and healthy fats can support sustained energy levels, cognitive function, and mood throughout the morning.

3. Strategic Snacking: Incorporating nutrient-dense snacks between meals can help maintain energy levels and prevent overeating at subsequent meals. Opt for snacks that combine carbohydrates with protein or healthy fats to provide sustained energy and promote feelings of fullness. Examples include fruit with nuts or yogurt, whole grain crackers with cheese, or vegetable sticks with hummus.

4. Meal Composition and Timing: The composition and timing of meals can influence energy levels and metabolism. Aim to consume larger meals earlier in the day when energy needs are

highest and spread out calories evenly throughout the day. Avoid heavy, high-fat meals close to bedtime, as they may disrupt sleep quality and digestion, leading to decreased energy levels the next day.

5. Hydration: Adequate hydration is essential for maintaining energy levels and supporting overall health. Dehydration can lead to fatigue, decreased cognitive function, and impaired physical performance. Aim to drink water throughout the day and consume hydrating foods such as fruits and vegetables to support optimal hydration and energy levels.

Conclusion:

Timing meals and snacks strategically throughout the day plays a vital role in sustaining energy levels, supporting metabolism, and promoting overall health and well-being. By prioritizing balanced meals and snacks that combine carbohydrates, proteins, and healthy fats, individuals can provide their bodies with the nutrients needed for sustained energy and optimal functioning. Consistency in meal timing and composition, along with adequate hydration, helps stabilize blood sugar levels, prevent energy dips, and support cognitive and physical performance throughout the day.

Resources:

1. Academy of Nutrition and Dietetics. "Timing Your Meals: Does It Really Matter When You Eat?" (https://www.eatright.org/health/weight-loss/healthy-eating/timing-your-meals-does-it-really-matter-when-you-eat)

2. Mayo Clinic.
"Eating and Exercise: 5 Tips to Maximize Your Workouts." (https://www.mayoclinic.org/healthy-lifestyle/fitness/in-depth/exercise/art-20045506)

3. Harvard Health Publishing. "The Nutrition Source - Healthy Eating Plate."

3.5 Balancing Macronutrients for Enhanced Energy

"Balance is not something you find, it's something you create." - Jana Kingsford

Introduction:

Balancing macronutrients—carbohydrates, proteins, and fats—in one's diet is crucial for sustaining energy levels, supporting metabolism, and promoting overall health and well-being. Each macronutrient plays a unique role in energy production and nutrient absorption, and achieving the right balance ensures optimal functioning of the body and mind. By understanding the roles of carbohydrates, proteins, and fats and how they interact to provide sustained energy, individuals can make informed dietary choices to enhance their energy levels and overall vitality.

Key Insights:

1. Carbohydrates for Immediate Energy: Carbohydrates are the body's primary source of energy, providing readily available fuel for physical activity and brain function. Simple carbohydrates, such as sugars and refined grains, are quickly digested and absorbed, providing a rapid but short-lived energy boost. Complex carbohydrates, found in whole grains, fruits, vegetables, and legumes, offer sustained energy due to their slower digestion and steady release of glucose into the bloodstream.

2. Proteins for Muscle Repair and Satiety: Proteins play essential roles in muscle repair, growth, and maintenance, as well as in hormone synthesis and immune function. Including protein-rich foods in meals and snacks helps stabilize blood sugar levels, promote feelings of fullness, and support muscle recovery after exercise. Sources of lean protein include poultry, fish, tofu, legumes, dairy products, and nuts.

3. Fats for Sustained Energy and Nutrient Absorption: Dietary fats are essential for energy production, providing a concentrated source of calories and serving as carriers for fat-soluble vitamins (A, D, E, and K). Healthy fats, such as monounsaturated and polyunsaturated fats found in avocados, nuts, seeds, and olive oil, support heart health, cognitive function, and satiety. Including a moderate amount of healthy fats in meals helps provide sustained energy and aids in the absorption of fat-soluble nutrients.

4. Balancing Macronutrients for Optimal Energy: Achieving a balance of carbohydrates, proteins, and fats in meals and snacks is key to maintaining stable energy levels throughout the day. The ideal macronutrient ratio may vary depending on individual factors such as age, gender, activity level, and health status. However, a general guideline is to aim for a balanced plate that includes a variety of nutrient-dense foods from all three macronutrient groups to support energy production, satiety, and overall health.

Conclusion:

Balancing macronutrients—carbohydrates, proteins, and fats—in one's diet is essential for sustaining energy levels, supporting metabolism, and promoting overall health and well-being. Each macronutrient plays a unique role in energy production, nutrient absorption, and satiety, and achieving the right balance ensures optimal functioning of the body and mind. By prioritizing nutrient-dense foods from all three macronutrient groups and making informed dietary choices, individuals can enhance their energy levels, improve their overall vitality, and support long-term health and well-being.

Resources:

1. Harvard T.H. Chan School of Public Health.
"The Nutrition Source - Healthy Eating Plate."
(https://www.hsph.harvard.edu/nutritionsource/healthy-eatin g-plate/)

2. Academy of Nutrition and Dietetics.
"Macronutrients: The Importance of Carbohydrate, Protein, and   Fat."
(https://www.eatright.org/food/nutrition/dietary-guidelines-a nd-myplate/macronutrients-the-importance-of-carbohydrate-p rotein-and-fat)

3. American Heart Association. "Know Your Fats."
(https://www.heart.org/en/healthy-living/healthy-eating/eat-s mart/fats/know-your-fats)

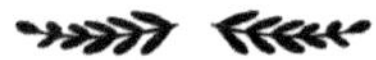

Nutrition for Mental Well-being

4.1 The Gut-Brain Connection: How Nutrition Affects Mood

"The food you eat can either be the safest and most powerful form of medicine, or the slowest form of poison." - Ann Wigmore

Introduction:

The gut-brain connection highlights the intricate relationship between the gastrointestinal system and mental health, emphasizing how nutrition influences mood, cognition, and emotional well-being. Emerging research suggests that the gut microbiota, the trillions of microorganisms residing in the digestive tract, play a pivotal role in regulating brain function and mental health. Understanding how nutrition affects the gut-brain axis offers insights into dietary strategies for promoting positive mood and emotional resilience.

Key Insights:

1. Microbiota Diversity and Mental Health: The gut microbiota composition influences neurotransmitter production, neuroinflammation, and stress response, all of which impact mood regulation and mental health. Imbalances in gut bacteria, known as dysbiosis, have been linked to mood disorders such as depression, anxiety, and stress-related conditions. Consuming a diverse range of plant-based foods, fiber-rich foods, and probiotics supports gut microbiota diversity and may contribute to improved mood and emotional well-being.

2. Nutrient Signaling and Brain Function: Nutrients derived from the diet, such as omega-3 fatty acids, vitamins, minerals, and phytonutrients, play essential roles in brain function and mood regulation. For example, omega-3 fatty acids found in fatty fish, flaxseeds, and walnuts are associated with reduced inflammation and improved mood. B-vitamins, particularly folate and B12, are crucial for neurotransmitter synthesis and may help alleviate symptoms of depression and anxiety.

3. Impact of Dietary Patterns on Mood: Dietary patterns, such as the Mediterranean diet and the DASH (Dietary Approaches to Stop Hypertension) diet, are associated with lower risk of depression and improved mental health outcomes. These diets emphasize whole, nutrient-dense foods such as fruits, vegetables, whole grains, lean proteins, and healthy fats, while limiting processed foods, sugars, and unhealthy fats. Adopting a dietary pattern rich in plant-based foods and antioxidants supports brain health and may enhance mood resilience.

4. Psychobiotics and Mood Modulation: Psychobiotics are live microorganisms that confer mental health benefits when consumed in adequate amounts. Probiotic-rich foods like yogurt, kefir, kimchi, and sauerkraut contain beneficial bacteria that may positively influence mood and stress response by modulating the gut microbiota. Prebiotic fibers found in fruits, vegetables, and whole grains serve as fuel for probiotics, further supporting gut health and emotional well-being.

Conclusion:

The gut-brain connection underscores the profound impact of nutrition on mood and mental health, highlighting the importance of adopting dietary strategies that support gut microbiota diversity, nutrient signaling, and emotional resilience. By prioritizing whole, nutrient-dense foods rich in fiber, omega-3 fatty acids, vitamins, and probiotics, individuals can optimize gut health, regulate mood, and promote overall well-being. Understanding the role of nutrition in the gut-brain axis empowers individuals to make informed dietary choices that nurture both their physical and mental health.

Resources:

1. Harvard Health Publishing. "The gut-brain connection." (https://www.health.harvard.edu/diseases-and-conditions/the-gut-brain-connection)

2. International Society for Nutritional Psychiatry Research. (https://www.isnpr.org/)

3. The American Journal of Clinical Nutrition. "Nutritional psychiatry: where to next?"

4.2 Foods that Boost Brain Health and Cognitive Function

"When you eat, appreciate every last bite. It's not just about the taste, but the experience." - Unknown

Introduction:

Foods that boost brain health and cognitive function play a crucial role in supporting mental clarity, memory, focus, and overall cognitive well-being. Research suggests that certain nutrients, antioxidants, and bioactive compounds found in various foods can protect brain cells, enhance neurotransmitter function, and promote neuroplasticity. Understanding the impact of dietary choices on brain health empowers individuals to make informed decisions to optimize cognitive function and maintain brain vitality throughout life.

Key Insights:

1. Omega-3 Fatty Acids: Omega-3 fatty acids, particularly EPA (eicosapentaenoic acid) and DHA (docosahexaenoic acid), are essential for brain health and cognitive function. Found abundantly in fatty fish such as salmon, mackerel, and sardines, as well as in walnuts, flaxseeds, and chia seeds, omega-3s support neuronal membrane integrity, reduce inflammation, and promote synaptic plasticity, enhancing learning and memory.

2. Antioxidant-Rich Foods: Antioxidants, such as vitamins C and E, beta-carotene, and flavonoids, help protect brain cells from oxidative stress and inflammation, which can contribute to cognitive decline and neurodegenerative diseases. Consuming a variety of antioxidant-rich foods, including berries, dark leafy greens, nuts, seeds, and colorful fruits and vegetables, supports brain health and may reduce the risk of age-related cognitive impairment.

3. Brain-Boosting Vitamins and Minerals: Certain vitamins and minerals are essential for optimal brain function and cognitive performance. Vitamin B12, found in animal products like meat, fish, eggs, and dairy, is crucial for nerve function and myelin synthesis, while folate, found in leafy greens, legumes, and fortified grains, supports neurotransmitter synthesis and methylation processes. Minerals such as iron, zinc, and magnesium also play roles in cognitive function and brain health.

4. Polyphenol-Rich Foods: Polyphenols are bioactive compounds found in plant foods that exhibit antioxidant and anti-inflammatory properties, supporting brain health and cognitive function. Foods rich in polyphenols include dark chocolate, green tea, red wine, berries, nuts, and spices like turmeric and cinnamon. Polyphenols may enhance neuronal communication, protect against age-related cognitive decline, and promote neurogenesis and synaptic plasticity.

Conclusion:

Foods that boost brain health and cognitive function are rich in omega-3 fatty acids, antioxidants, vitamins, minerals, and polyphenols, all of which support neuronal integrity, neurotransmitter function, and cognitive performance. By incorporating a variety of brain-boosting foods into their diet, individuals can nourish their brains, protect against cognitive decline, and promote lifelong cognitive vitality. Understanding the impact of dietary choices on brain health empowers individuals to prioritize foods that support cognitive function and overall well-being.

Resources:

1. Alzheimer's Association. "Brain Health & Your Diet." (https://www.alz.org/alzheimers-dementia/research_progress/ prevention/brain-health)

2. Harvard Health Publishing.
"Nutritional strategies to boost brain power." (https://www.health.harvard.edu/mind-and-mood/nutritional -strategies-to-boost-brain-power)

3. National Institute on Aging.
"Eat Smart for a Healthier Brain." (https://www.nia.nih.gov/health/eat-smart-healthier-brain)

4. American Heart Association. "Healthy Eating: Eat Smart."

4.3 Omega-3 Fatty Acids and Their Role in Mental Well-being

"Every time you eat is an opportunity to nourish your body and soul." - Unknown

Introduction:

Omega-3 fatty acids, particularly EPA (eicosapentaenoic acid) and DHA (docosahexaenoic acid), are essential nutrients with a profound impact on mental well-being. Research suggests that omega-3s play crucial roles in brain development, neurotransmitter function, and neuroinflammation regulation, making them vital for cognitive function, mood regulation, and overall mental health. Understanding the role of omega-3 fatty acids in mental well-being sheds light on the importance of incorporating these nutrients into one's diet to support emotional resilience and psychological vitality.

Key Insights:

1. Neurotransmitter Function: Omega-3 fatty acids are integral components of neuronal membranes and play essential roles in neurotransmitter signaling. DHA, in particular, is highly concentrated in the brain and retina and is involved in synaptic transmission, neuroplasticity, and neuronal membrane fluidity. Adequate intake of omega-3s supports optimal neurotransmitter function, enhancing mood regulation and cognitive performance.

2. Anti-inflammatory Properties: Chronic inflammation in the brain has been implicated in the pathogenesis of mood disorders such as depression and anxiety. Omega-3 fatty acids

exert anti-inflammatory effects by inhibiting pro-inflammatory cytokines and modulating immune responses, thereby reducing neuroinflammation and oxidative stress. By mitigating neuroinflammation, omega-3s may help alleviate symptoms of depression and support mental well-being.

3. Neuroprotective Effects: Omega-3 fatty acids possess neuroprotective properties, safeguarding against neuronal damage and degeneration. EPA and DHA promote neuronal survival, enhance synaptic plasticity, and stimulate neurotrophic factor expression, supporting neurogenesis and neuronal repair processes. These neuroprotective effects may contribute to improved mood, cognition, and resilience to stress and adversity.

4. Clinical Evidence: Numerous clinical studies have investigated the impact of omega-3 supplementation on mental health outcomes, particularly in the context of depression, anxiety, and mood disorders. While results have been mixed, meta-analyses suggest that omega-3 supplementation, particularly with higher doses of EPA, may be beneficial for reducing depressive symptoms and improving treatment response in individuals with depression. Additionally, omega-3s may have a protective effect against cognitive decline and age-related cognitive impairment.

Conclusion:

Omega-3 fatty acids play a crucial role in mental well-being, supporting neurotransmitter function, neuroinflammation regulation, and neuroprotection. Incorporating omega-3-rich foods such as fatty fish, flaxseeds, chia seeds, and walnuts into one's diet, or supplementing with high-quality fish oil, can help ensure an adequate intake of these essential nutrients. By nourishing the brain with omega-3 fatty acids, individuals can support cognitive function, mood regulation, and emotional resilience, promoting overall mental well-being and vitality.

Resources:

1. National Institutes of Health (NIH). "Omega-3 Fatty Acids: Fact Sheet for Health Professionals." (https://ods.od.nih.gov/factsheets/Omega3FattyAcids-Health Professional/)

2. American Psychological Association. "The Connection Between Omega-3 Fatty Acids and Depression." (https://www.apa.org/monitor/2015/03/cover-oil)

3. Harvard Health Publishing.
"The brain and omega-3 fatty acids." (https://www.health.harvard.edu/blog/omega-3-fatty-acids-for -mood-disorders-2018080314414)

4.4 The Influence of Sugar and Processed Foods on Mental Health

"Eating mindfully is a way to deepen our understanding of ourselves and our relationship to the world." - Jan Chozen Bays

Introduction:

The influence of sugar and processed foods on mental health is a topic of growing interest, as dietary patterns have been increasingly linked to mood disorders, cognitive function, and overall mental well-being. Sugar and processed foods are ubiquitous in modern diets, yet their high consumption has been associated with adverse effects on mental health, including increased risk of depression, anxiety, and impaired cognitive function. Understanding the impact of sugar and processed foods on mental health is essential for promoting optimal psychological well-being and preventing mental health disorders.

Key Insights:

1. Blood Sugar Dysregulation: Consumption of sugary and processed foods can lead to rapid spikes and subsequent crashes

in blood sugar levels, contributing to fluctuations in mood and energy levels. High-glycemic foods, such as sugary snacks, sodas, and refined grains, cause rapid increases in blood glucose followed by insulin surges, which may exacerbate feelings of anxiety, irritability, and fatigue.

2. Inflammation and Oxidative Stress: Diets high in sugar and processed foods are associated with chronic low-grade inflammation and oxidative stress, which have been implicated in the pathogenesis of mood disorders such as depression and anxiety. Excessive sugar intake promotes the release of pro-inflammatory cytokines and reactive oxygen species, contributing to neuroinflammation and neuronal damage in the brain.

3. Gut-Brain Axis Dysfunction: Sugar and processed foods can disrupt the delicate balance of the gut microbiota, leading to dysbiosis and alterations in gut-brain communication. Imbalances in gut bacteria have been linked to mood disorders and cognitive dysfunction, as the gut microbiota produce neurotransmitters and modulate neuroinflammatory pathways that influence mood and behavior.

4. Nutrient Deficiencies: Diets high in sugar and processed foods often lack essential nutrients critical for mental health, including omega-3 fatty acids, vitamins, minerals, and antioxidants. Inadequate intake of these nutrients, coupled with increased consumption of sugary and processed foods,

may impair neurotransmitter synthesis, neuronal function, and neuroprotection, predisposing individuals to mood disorders and cognitive decline.

Conclusion:

The influence of sugar and processed foods on mental health extends beyond mere nutritional considerations, encompassing neurobiological, inflammatory, and gut-brain axis mechanisms. By recognizing the detrimental effects of excessive sugar and processed food consumption on mood, cognition, and overall mental well-being, individuals can make informed dietary choices to prioritize whole, nutrient-dense foods that support optimal mental health. Promoting a diet rich in fruits, vegetables, whole grains, lean proteins, and healthy fats while minimizing intake of sugary and processed foods can help protect against mood disorders, enhance cognitive function, and foster resilience to stress.

Resources:

1. Harvard Health Publishing.
"Nutritional psychiatry: Your brain on food." (https://www.health.harvard.edu/blog/nutritional-psychiatry-your-brain-on-food-201511168626)

2. National Institutes of Health (NIH). "Dietary sugars and mental health: A systematic review

of prospective and randomized controlled studies."
(https://www.ncbi.nlm.nih.gov/pmc/articles/PMC6146353/)

3. American Psychological Association. "The link between diet and mental health." (https://www.apa.org/monitor/2017/09/food-mental-health)

4. World Health Organization (WHO). "Nutrition, health, and mental well-being."

4.5 Mindful Eating Practices for Emotional Well-being

"The gift of learning to meditate is the greatest gift you can give yourself in this lifetime." - Sogyal Rinpoche

Introduction:

Mindful eating practices involve cultivating awareness and non-judgmental attention to the present moment while consuming food. These practices encourage individuals to tune into their physical hunger and satiety cues, as well as the sensory experiences of eating, such as taste, texture, and aroma. Mindful eating has gained recognition for its potential to promote emotional well-being by fostering a healthier relationship with food, reducing stress-related eating behaviors, and enhancing overall satisfaction with meals. Understanding and implementing mindful eating practices can contribute to improved emotional resilience, greater self-awareness, and a more positive relationship with food and body.

Key Insights:

1. Awareness of Hunger and Fullness: Mindful eating emphasizes tuning into internal hunger and fullness cues to guide eating behaviors. By pausing to assess physical hunger before eating and paying attention to satiety signals during meals, individuals can prevent overeating, promote a sense of satisfaction, and develop a greater trust in their body's innate wisdom to regulate food intake.

2. Attentive Eating: Mindful eating involves slowing down and savoring each bite of food, engaging all the senses to fully experience the tastes, textures, and aromas of the meal. By practicing attentive eating, individuals can cultivate a deeper appreciation for food, enhance the pleasure of eating, and reduce the tendency to consume food mindlessly or impulsively in response to emotional cues.

3. Non-judgmental Awareness: Mindful eating encourages non-judgmental awareness of thoughts, feelings, and sensations that arise during eating, without assigning value or criticism. By observing and accepting experiences without judgment,

individuals can develop greater self-awareness, identify emotional triggers for eating, and cultivate a compassionate attitude toward themselves and their eating behaviors.

4. Emotional Regulation: Mindful eating practices can help individuals become more attuned to their emotional states and the ways in which emotions influence eating behaviors. Rather than using food as a primary coping mechanism for stress, anxiety, or boredom, individuals can develop alternative strategies for emotional regulation, such as mindfulness, deep breathing, or engaging in enjoyable activities that nourish the soul without relying on food.

Conclusion:

Mindful eating practices offer a holistic approach to promoting emotional well-being by fostering a more conscious, intentional, and balanced relationship with food. By cultivating awareness, attention, and non-judgmental acceptance during eating, individuals can develop healthier eating habits, reduce stress-related eating behaviors, and enhance their overall satisfaction with meals. Incorporating mindful eating into daily life can contribute to greater emotional resilience, improved self-regulation, and a deeper sense of connection with oneself and the present moment.

Resources:

1. The Center for Mindful Eating. (https://www.thecenterformindfuleating.org/)

2. Mindful.org. "Mindful Eating." (https://www.mindful.org/category/food/)

3. Harvard Health Publishing. "8 steps to mindful eating." (https://www.health.harvard.edu/staying-healthy/8-steps-to-mindful-eating)

4. The American Heart Association. "Mindful Eating." (https://www.heart.org/en/healthy-living/healthy-eating/eat-smart/nutrition-basics/mindful-eating)

Eating for Longevity

5.1 Exploring Anti-inflammatory Foods and Their Benefits

"Eat the rainbow for vibrant health and longevity."
- Unknown

Introduction:

Exploring anti-inflammatory foods and their benefits is essential in understanding the role of diet in promoting overall health and reducing the risk of chronic diseases associated with inflammation. Chronic inflammation is implicated in the pathogenesis of various conditions, including cardiovascular disease, diabetes, arthritis, and certain cancers. Anti-inflammatory foods contain bioactive compounds that help modulate inflammatory pathways, reduce oxidative stress, and support immune function. By incorporating these foods into one's diet, individuals can potentially mitigate inflammation, promote tissue repair, and enhance overall well-being.

Key Insights:

1. Rich in Phytonutrients: Anti-inflammatory foods are rich in phytonutrients, including polyphenols, flavonoids, carotenoids, and antioxidants, which possess potent anti-inflammatory properties. These bioactive compounds scavenge free radicals, inhibit pro-inflammatory enzymes, and regulate immune responses, thereby reducing inflammation and oxidative damage in the body.

2. Omega-3 Fatty Acids: Omega-3 fatty acids, particularly EPA (eicosapentaenoic acid) and DHA (docosahexaenoic acid), are well-known for their anti-inflammatory effects. Found abundantly in fatty fish such as salmon, mackerel, and sardines, as well as in flaxseeds, chia seeds, and walnuts, omega-3s help counteract the pro-inflammatory actions of omega-6 fatty acids and promote the synthesis of anti-inflammatory lipid mediators.

3. Whole Plant Foods: Whole plant foods, such as fruits, vegetables, legumes, nuts, and seeds, are foundational components of an anti-inflammatory diet. These foods are high in fiber, vitamins, minerals, and phytonutrients, which collectively exert anti-inflammatory effects and support overall

health. Incorporating a variety of colorful fruits and vegetables into meals ensures a diverse array of phytonutrients with unique anti-inflammatory properties.

4. Herbs and Spices: Herbs and spices are potent sources of anti-inflammatory compounds that can be easily incorporated into cooking. Turmeric, ginger, cinnamon, garlic, and rosemary are examples of culinary herbs and spices with demonstrated anti-inflammatory properties. These ingredients contain bioactive compounds such as curcumin, gingerol, cinnamaldehyde, allicin, and rosmarinic acid, which possess antioxidant, anti-inflammatory, and immune-modulating effects.

Conclusion:

Exploring anti-inflammatory foods and their benefits provides valuable insights into the role of nutrition in modulating inflammation and promoting overall health. By incorporating a diverse array of anti-inflammatory foods into one's diet, individuals can harness the power of phytonutrients, omega-3 fatty acids, whole plant foods, and culinary herbs and spices to mitigate chronic inflammation, reduce the risk of chronic diseases, and enhance overall well-being. Embracing an anti-inflammatory diet as part of a healthy lifestyle can serve as a proactive approach to supporting immune function, optimizing health outcomes, and fostering longevity.

Resources:

1. Arthritis Foundation. "The Ultimate Arthritis Diet." [Link](https://www.arthritis.org/health-wellness/healthy-living/nutrition/anti-inflammatory/the-arthritis-diet)

2. Harvard Health Publishing. "Foods that fight inflammation." [Link](https://www.health.harvard.edu/staying-healthy/foods-that-fight-inflammation)

3. Cleveland Clinic. "Anti-Inflammatory Diet: How to Choose the Right Cooking Oils." [Link](https://health.clevelandclinic.org/anti-inflammatory-diet-how-to-choose-the-right-cooking-oils/)

4. The Institute for Functional Medicine. "The Anti-Inflammatory Diet." [Link]()

5.2 The Mediterranean Diet: A Blueprint for Longevity

"The Mediterranean diet is more than just a diet—it's a lifestyle rooted in tradition, culture, and connection to the land and sea." - Unknown

Introduction:

The Mediterranean diet, inspired by the traditional dietary patterns of countries bordering the Mediterranean Sea, has garnered widespread recognition as a blueprint for longevity and overall well-being. Characterized by an abundance of fruits, vegetables, whole grains, legumes, nuts, seeds, olive oil, and moderate consumption of fish, poultry, dairy, and red wine, the Mediterranean diet offers a holistic approach to promoting health and longevity. Research suggests that adherence to the Mediterranean diet is associated with numerous health benefits, including reduced risk of chronic diseases, improved cardiovascular health, enhanced cognitive function, and increased longevity. Exploring the principles and benefits of the Mediterranean diet provides valuable insights into its role as a sustainable and culturally rich dietary pattern conducive to longevity and vitality.

Key Insights:

1. Plant-Centered Eating: The Mediterranean diet emphasizes plant-centered eating, with fruits, vegetables, whole grains, legumes, nuts, and seeds forming the foundation of meals. These plant-based foods are rich in fiber, vitamins, minerals, and phytonutrients, which contribute to overall health, support digestive function, and provide essential nutrients for vitality and longevity.

2. Healthy Fats: Unlike conventional Western diets high in saturated and trans fats, the Mediterranean diet prioritizes healthy fats, particularly monounsaturated fats found in olive oil, nuts, and avocados. These fats are associated with reduced inflammation, improved cholesterol levels, and enhanced cardiovascular health, all of which contribute to longevity and disease prevention.

3. Moderate Fish and Poultry: The Mediterranean diet includes moderate consumption of fish, poultry, and eggs, which provide high-quality protein, essential amino acids, and omega-3 fatty acids. Fish, especially fatty varieties like salmon, sardines, and mackerel, are rich in omega-3s, which have anti-inflammatory properties and are associated with reduced risk of heart disease and cognitive decline.

4. Red Wine in Moderation: Moderate consumption of red wine, particularly with meals, is a hallmark of the Mediterranean diet. Red wine contains polyphenols, such as resveratrol, which exhibit antioxidant and anti-inflammatory effects. Consuming red wine in moderation has been associated with improved cardiovascular health and longevity, although excessive alcohol intake should be avoided.

Conclusion:

The Mediterranean diet offers a sustainable and culturally rich approach to promoting health, longevity, and overall well-being.

By prioritizing whole, minimally processed foods such as fruits, vegetables, whole grains, legumes, nuts, seeds, and olive oil, while incorporating moderate amounts of fish, poultry, dairy, and red wine, individuals can embrace a dietary pattern that nourishes the body, supports longevity, and fosters a deep appreciation for food, community, and life. Embracing the principles of the Mediterranean diet as a blueprint for longevity provides a holistic framework for optimizing health outcomes, enhancing vitality, and savoring the pleasures of food and life.

Resources:

1. Oldways. "Mediterranean Diet Pyramid." [Link](https://oldwayspt.org/traditional-diets/mediterranean-diet)

2. Mayo Clinic.
"Mediterranean diet: A heart-healthy eating plan." [Link](https://www.mayoclinic.org/healthy-lifestyle/nutrition-and-healthy-eating/in-depth/mediterranean-diet/art-20047801)

3. Harvard T.H. Chan School of Public Health.
"The Nutrition Source - The Mediterranean Diet." [Link](https://www.hsph.harvard.edu/nutritionsource/healthy-eating-plate/)

4. American Heart Association. "Mediterranean Diet." [Link]()

5.3 Superfoods for Longevity and Disease Prevention

"The richness of our health depends on the diversity of our diet." - Unknown

Introduction:

Superfoods, nutrient-dense foods rich in vitamins, minerals, antioxidants, and phytonutrients, have gained widespread attention for their potential to promote longevity and prevent chronic diseases. Incorporating superfoods into one's diet can provide a multitude of health benefits, including reducing inflammation, supporting immune function, enhancing cardiovascular health, and protecting against oxidative stress. By prioritizing the consumption of superfoods as part of a balanced diet, individuals can optimize their nutritional intake, mitigate the risk of age-related diseases, and foster overall well-being. Exploring the role of superfoods in longevity and disease prevention offers valuable insights into dietary strategies for promoting healthspan and vitality.

Key Insights:

1. Colorful Fruits and Vegetables: Colorful fruits and vegetables, such as berries, leafy greens, cruciferous vegetables, and citrus fruits, are rich in vitamins, minerals, and antioxidants that combat oxidative stress and inflammation. These superfoods contain phytonutrients like flavonoids, carotenoids, and polyphenols, which support cellular health, enhance immune function, and reduce the risk of chronic diseases, including cancer, heart disease, and neurodegenerative disorders.

2. Omega-3-Rich Foods: Omega-3 fatty acids, found in fatty fish (e.g., salmon, mackerel, sardines), flaxseeds, chia seeds, and walnuts, are potent superfoods with anti-inflammatory properties. Omega-3s support cardiovascular health, brain function, and joint health, and may reduce the risk of age-related cognitive decline and inflammatory conditions such as arthritis.

3. Legumes and Pulses: Legumes and pulses, including beans, lentils, chickpeas, and peas, are nutritional powerhouses rich in fiber, protein, vitamins, and minerals. These superfoods promote satiety, stabilize blood sugar levels, and support digestive health. Regular consumption of legumes is associated with reduced risk of cardiovascular disease, type 2 diabetes, and certain cancers.

4. Nuts and Seeds: Nuts and seeds, such as almonds, walnuts, chia seeds, and flaxseeds, are concentrated sources of healthy fats,

protein, fiber, vitamins, and minerals. These superfoods provide essential nutrients for heart health, brain function, and overall vitality. Incorporating nuts and seeds into the diet may help lower cholesterol levels, improve blood sugar control, and reduce inflammation.

Conclusion:

Superfoods play a pivotal role in promoting longevity and preventing chronic diseases by supplying essential nutrients, antioxidants, and bioactive compounds that support overall health and well-being. By incorporating a diverse array of superfoods into one's diet, individuals can optimize their nutritional intake, mitigate inflammation, and protect against age-related diseases. Prioritizing the consumption of colorful fruits and vegetables, omega-3-rich foods, legumes and pulses, nuts, and seeds provides a foundation for optimal healthspan, vitality, and disease prevention. Embracing superfoods as part of a balanced diet offers a proactive approach to enhancing quality of life and fostering lifelong well-being.

Resources:

1. Harvard T.H. Chan School of Public Health. "Superfoods or Superhype?" [Link](https://www.hsph.harvard.edu/nutritionsource/superfoods/)

2. Cleveland Clinic. "10 Superfoods to Add to Your Diet." [Link](https://health.clevelandclinic.org/10-superfoods-to-add-to-your-diet/)

3. Mayo Clinic. "Nutrition basics: Superfoods to boost your health." [Link](https://www.mayoclinic.org/healthy-lifestyle/nutrition-and-healthy-eating/expert-answers/superfoods/faq-20057899)

4. National Institutes of Health (NIH). "Superfoods: Health or Hype?" [Link]()

5.4 Incorporating Antioxidants for Cellular Health

"To keep the body in good health is a duty... otherwise, we shall not be able to keep our mind strong and clear." - Buddha

Introduction:

Incorporating antioxidants into the diet is essential for supporting cellular health and overall well-being. Antioxidants are compounds that neutralize harmful free radicals, reactive molecules that can damage cells and contribute to oxidative stress, inflammation, and aging. By consuming a variety of antioxidant-rich foods, individuals can protect cells from oxidative damage, enhance immune function, and reduce the risk of chronic diseases. Understanding the importance of antioxidants for cellular health provides valuable insights into dietary strategies for promoting longevity and vitality.

Key Insights:

1. Types of Antioxidants: Antioxidants encompass a diverse range of compounds, including vitamins (e.g., vitamin C, vitamin E), minerals (e.g., selenium, zinc), phytonutrients (e.g., flavonoids, carotenoids), and enzymes (e.g., superoxide dismutase, catalase). Each antioxidant exerts unique protective effects on cells and tissues, scavenging free radicals and preventing oxidative damage.

2. Foods Rich in Antioxidants: Incorporating antioxidant-rich foods into the diet is key to supporting cellular health. Colorful fruits and vegetables, such as berries, citrus fruits, leafy greens, tomatoes, and bell peppers, are excellent sources of vitamins C and E, as well as phytonutrients like flavonoids and carotenoids. Other antioxidant-rich foods include nuts, seeds, whole grains, legumes, and spices like turmeric and cinnamon.

3. Synergistic Effects: Antioxidants work synergistically to protect cells from oxidative stress, amplifying their collective antioxidant capacity. For example, vitamin C regenerates vitamin E after it has neutralized a free radical, while

polyphenols in fruits and vegetables enhance the activity of endogenous antioxidants enzymes. Consuming a diverse array of antioxidant-rich foods ensures a synergistic blend of antioxidants to support cellular health.

4. Long-Term Benefits: Regular consumption of antioxidants has been associated with numerous health benefits, including reduced risk of chronic diseases such as cardiovascular disease, cancer, and neurodegenerative disorders. Antioxidants support immune function, promote skin health, and may slow the aging process by protecting cells from damage caused by environmental toxins, UV radiation, and other stressors.

Conclusion:

Incorporating antioxidants into the diet is essential for maintaining cellular health, supporting immune function, and reducing the risk of chronic diseases associated with oxidative stress and inflammation. By consuming a diverse array of antioxidant-rich foods, individuals can protect cells from damage, enhance overall well-being, and promote longevity. Prioritizing fruits, vegetables, nuts, seeds, whole grains, and spices as part of a balanced diet provides a natural and effective approach to incorporating antioxidants for cellular health and vitality.

Resources:

1. Harvard T.H. Chan School of Public Health. "Antioxidants: Beyond the Hype." [Link](https://www.hsph.harvard.edu/nutritionsource/antioxidants/)

2. National Institutes of Health (NIH). "Antioxidants: In Depth." [Link](https://www.nccih.nih.gov/health/antioxidants-in-depth)

3. American Heart Association. "Antioxidants in the Diet." [Link](https://www.heart.org/en/healthy-living/healthy-eating/eat-smart/nutrition-basics/antioxidants-in-the-diet)

4. Cleveland Clinic. "The Best Foods High in Antioxidants." [Link]()

5.5 The Role of Phytonutrients in Promoting Longevity

"Eat food. Not too much. Mostly plants." - Michael Pollan

Introduction:

Phytonutrients, natural compounds found in plants, play a significant role in promoting longevity and overall health. These bioactive substances contribute to the vibrant colors, flavors, and aromas of fruits, vegetables, herbs, spices, nuts, seeds, and whole grains. Phytonutrients possess potent antioxidant, anti-inflammatory, anti-cancer, and immune-modulating properties, which support cellular health, protect against chronic diseases, and enhance longevity. Understanding the role of phytonutrients in promoting longevity sheds light on the importance of incorporating a diverse array of plant-based foods into the diet to optimize healthspan and quality of life.

Key Insights:

1. Antioxidant Activity: Many phytonutrients act as antioxidants, scavenging free radicals and reactive oxygen species that can damage cells and contribute to aging and disease. Examples of antioxidant phytonutrients include flavonoids, polyphenols, carotenoids, and anthocyanins, which are abundant in fruits, vegetables, and herbs. By neutralizing oxidative stress, phytonutrients help protect cells from damage and support overall cellular health.

2. Anti-inflammatory Effects: Phytonutrients possess anti-inflammatory properties that help mitigate chronic inflammation, a key driver of age-related diseases such as cardiovascular disease, diabetes, and neurodegenerative disorders. Compounds like curcumin in turmeric, resveratrol in grapes, and quercetin in onions exert anti-inflammatory effects by modulating inflammatory pathways and reducing the production of inflammatory mediators.

3. Cellular Protection: Phytonutrients promote cellular health by enhancing the body's defense mechanisms against oxidative damage, DNA mutations, and cellular dysfunction. Certain phytonutrients, such as sulforaphane in cruciferous vegetables and epigallocatechin gallate (EGCG) in green tea, have been shown to activate cellular detoxification pathways, inhibit carcinogenesis, and promote apoptosis (programmed cell death) in cancer cells.

4. Cardiovascular Health: Many phytonutrients support cardiovascular health by reducing risk factors for heart disease, such as high cholesterol, hypertension, and inflammation. For example, flavonoids in cocoa, tea, and berries have been associated with improved endothelial function, reduced arterial stiffness, and lowered blood pressure, while polyphenols in red wine may help prevent atherosclerosis and improve blood lipid profiles.

Conclusion:

Phytonutrients play a crucial role in promoting longevity and enhancing overall health by supporting cellular function, reducing inflammation, and protecting against chronic diseases. Incorporating a diverse array of phytonutrient-rich plant-based foods into the diet, including fruits, vegetables, herbs, spices, nuts, seeds, and whole grains, provides an abundance of bioactive compounds that support vitality and well-being. By embracing a plant-centric dietary pattern rich in phytonutrients, individuals can optimize healthspan, reduce the risk of age-related diseases, and foster a vibrant and resilient body throughout life.

Resources:

1. National Institutes of Health (NIH). "Phytonutrients." [Link](https://ods.od.nih.gov/factsheets/Phytonutrients-HealthProfessional/)

2. Harvard T.H. Chan School of Public Health.
"The Nutrition Source - Phytonutrients." [Link](https://www.hsph.harvard.edu/nutritionsource/phytonutrients/)

3. Cleveland Clinic.
"Phytonutrients: Paint your plate with the colors of the rainbow."

[Link](https://health.clevelandclinic.org/phytonutrients-paint-your-plate-with-the-colors-of-the-rainbow/)

4. American Institute for Cancer Research (AICR). "Phytochemicals and the Cancer Fighting Diet." [Link](https://www.aicr.org/resources/blog/phytochemicals-and-the-cancer-fighting-diet/)

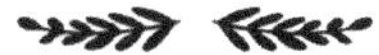

Practical Tips for Vibrant Eating

6.1 Meal Planning Strategies for Nutritious Eating

"Failing to plan is planning to fail." - Alan Lakein

Introduction:

Meal planning strategies are essential tools for promoting nutritious eating habits and supporting overall health and well-being. By taking a proactive approach to meal planning, individuals can ensure that their diets are balanced, varied, and nutrient-dense, while also saving time, reducing food waste, and minimizing reliance on convenience foods. Implementing effective meal planning strategies involves thoughtful consideration of dietary preferences, nutritional needs, cooking skills, and lifestyle factors. Exploring meal planning strategies for nutritious eating provides valuable insights into practical approaches for optimizing dietary intake and fostering long-term health.

Key Insights:

1. Assessment of Dietary Needs: Effective meal planning begins with an assessment of individual dietary needs, preferences, and goals. Consider factors such as age, gender, activity level, food allergies or intolerances, cultural or religious practices, and health conditions when designing meal plans. Tailoring meal plans to meet specific nutritional requirements ensures that individuals receive adequate nutrients to support optimal health and performance.

2. Balanced Macronutrient Distribution: A well-balanced meal plan includes a variety of macronutrients—carbohydrates, proteins, and fats—in appropriate proportions to meet energy needs and promote satiety. Aim to incorporate whole grains, lean proteins, healthy fats, and a variety of fruits and vegetables into meals to ensure a diverse array of nutrients and phytochemicals.

3. Incorporation of Variety and Diversity: Emphasize variety and diversity in meal planning to maximize nutritional intake and enjoyment of meals. Rotate through different food

groups, cooking methods, flavors, and cuisines to keep meals interesting and prevent dietary monotony. Experiment with new ingredients, recipes, and cultural dishes to expand culinary horizons and discover new flavors and textures.

4. Preparation and Organization: Successful meal planning relies on preparation and organization to streamline the cooking process and facilitate adherence to healthy eating goals. Set aside dedicated time each week for meal planning, grocery shopping, and meal prep. Batch cooking, prepping ingredients in advance, and utilizing time-saving kitchen gadgets can help make meal preparation more efficient and enjoyable.

Conclusion:

Meal planning strategies are invaluable tools for promoting nutritious eating habits, supporting health goals, and simplifying mealtime decisions. By adopting proactive meal planning practices, individuals can ensure that their diets are well-balanced, varied, and nutrient-rich, while also saving time, reducing stress, and minimizing food waste. Incorporating assessment of dietary needs, balanced macronutrient distribution, variety and diversity, and preparation and organization into meal planning efforts provides a solid foundation for achieving long-term success in maintaining a healthy lifestyle.

Resources:

1. Academy of Nutrition and Dietetics. "Meal Planning for Healthy Eating." (https://www.eatright.org/food/planning-and-prep/basic-meal -planning)

2. American Heart Association. "Healthy Eating on a Budget." (https://www.heart.org/en/healthy-living/healthy-eating/eat-s mart/nutrition-basics/healthy-eating-on-a-budget)

3. USDA ChooseMyPlate. "MyPlate Meal Planning." (https://www.choosemyplate.gov/eathealthy/MyPlate-Makeov er)

4. Cooking Light. "10 Essential Tips for Healthy Meal Planning."

6.2 Smart Grocery Shopping: Reading Labels and Making Healthy Choices

"Those who think they have no time for healthy eating will sooner or later have to find time for illness." - Edward Stanley

Introduction:

Smart grocery shopping is a cornerstone of maintaining a healthy diet and lifestyle. By learning to read labels and make informed choices, individuals can select nutritious foods that support their health goals, while also navigating the array of products available in supermarkets. Understanding how to interpret nutrition labels, ingredient lists, and health claims empowers consumers to make smarter choices and prioritize foods that contribute to overall well-being. Exploring strategies for smart grocery shopping provides valuable insights into making informed decisions and fostering healthier eating habits.

Key Insights:

1. Nutrition Label Reading: Nutrition labels provide valuable information about the nutrient content of packaged foods, including serving size, calories, macronutrients (such as carbohydrates, protein, and fat), and micronutrients (such as vitamins and minerals). Pay attention to portion sizes and serving sizes when interpreting nutrition labels, and aim to select foods that are lower in added sugars, saturated fats, and sodium.

2. Ingredient List Examination: The ingredient list on food labels provides insight into the composition of a product and can help consumers identify hidden additives, preservatives, and artificial ingredients. Look for foods with shorter ingredient lists

that contain recognizable, whole food ingredients, such as fruits, vegetables, whole grains, and lean proteins. Avoid products with long lists of additives, artificial colors, flavors, and sweeteners.

3. Health Claims Evaluation: Be discerning when evaluating health claims on food packaging, as these claims can be misleading or exaggerated. Terms like "all-natural," "organic," "low-fat," and "gluten-free" may not necessarily indicate a healthier choice. Instead, focus on the overall nutrient profile of the product, paying attention to key nutrients like fiber, vitamins, and minerals, as well as the presence of added sugars and unhealthy fats.

4. Strategic Shopping Strategies: Plan ahead and create a shopping list based on meal plans and dietary goals to avoid impulse purchases and unnecessary spending. Shop the perimeter of the grocery store, where fresh produce, lean proteins, dairy, and whole grains are typically located. Be selective when navigating the inner aisles, where processed and packaged foods are often displayed, and opt for minimally processed options whenever possible.

Conclusion:

Smart grocery shopping is a fundamental aspect of maintaining a healthy diet and lifestyle. By mastering the art of reading labels and making informed choices, individuals can select nutritious foods that align with their health goals and preferences. By prioritizing whole, minimally processed foods, paying attention to ingredient lists and nutrition labels, and critically evaluating health claims, consumers can navigate the supermarket aisles with confidence and make choices that support their well-being.

Resources:

1. American Heart Association. "Understanding Food Labels." (https://www.heart.org/en/healthy-living/healthy-eating/eat-smart/nutrition-basics/understanding-food-nutrition-labels)

2. EatRight.org. "How to Read a Nutrition Label." (https://www.eatright.org/food/nutrition/nutrition-facts-and-food-labels/how-to-read-a-nutrition-facts-label)

3. Mayo Clinic. "Nutrition Basics: Decoding Food Labels." (https://www.mayoclinic.org/healthy-lifestyle/nutrition-and-healthy-eating/in-depth/nutrition-basics/art-20045536)

4. Healthline. "How to Read Food Labels Without Being Tricked."

6.3 Tips for Eating Out: Making Healthier Choices at Restaurants

*"Eating out does not have to mean sacrificing health.
With mindful choices and strategic approaches,*

individuals can enjoy dining out while
still prioritizing nutrition and well-being." -
Unknown

Introduction:

Eating out at restaurants can present challenges to maintaining a healthy diet, as many menu options are often high in calories, saturated fats, sodium, and added sugars. However, with mindful choices and strategic approaches, individuals can enjoy dining out while still making healthier choices that align with their dietary goals. Understanding how to navigate restaurant menus, portion sizes, and cooking methods empowers individuals to make informed choices that prioritize nutrition and well-being. Exploring tips for eating out provides valuable insights into making healthier choices and promoting overall health when dining at restaurants.

Key Insights:

1. Review Menus Ahead of Time: Before dining out, take the time to review restaurant menus online, if available. Look for healthier options such as grilled or baked dishes, salads with lean proteins, and vegetable-based entrées. Planning your meal in advance can help you make healthier choices and avoid impulse decisions when faced with tempting menu items.

2. Choose Wisely: Opt for dishes that are prepared using healthier cooking methods, such as grilling, baking, steaming, or broiling, rather than fried or deep-fried options. Look for menu items that feature lean proteins like chicken, fish, or tofu, and incorporate plenty of vegetables. Be cautious of high-calorie toppings, dressings, and sauces, and ask for them on the side or for lighter alternatives.

3. Control Portion Sizes: Restaurant portions are often larger than what you would typically eat at home, leading to overconsumption of calories and nutrients. To control portion sizes, consider sharing an entrée with a dining companion or ask for a half portion. Alternatively, pack up half of your meal to take home for later, or order appetizers or starters instead of a full entrée.

4. Mindful Eating Practices: Practice mindful eating by paying attention to hunger and fullness cues, eating slowly, and savoring each bite. Focus on enjoying the flavors, textures, and aromas of your meal, rather than mindlessly consuming food. Pause between bites, and check in with yourself to assess your level of satisfaction and fullness.

Conclusion:

Making healthier choices when eating out at restaurants is entirely achievable with thoughtful planning and mindful decision-making. By reviewing menus ahead of time, choosing wisely, controlling portion sizes, and practicing mindful eating, individuals can navigate restaurant dining with confidence and support their health goals. By prioritizing nutrient-dense options, healthier cooking methods, and portion control, individuals can enjoy dining out while still making choices that contribute to their overall well-being.

Resources:

1. American Heart Association. "Eat Smart: Eating Out." (https://www.heart.org/en/healthy-living/healthy-eating/eat-smart/nutrition-basics/eating-out)

2. Centers for Disease Control and Prevention (CDC). "Making Healthier Choices at Restaurants." (https://www.cdc.gov/healthyweight/healthy_eating/restaurants.html)

3. Mayo Clinic. "Nutrition and Healthy Eating: Dining out? Think about your choices." (https://www.mayoclinic.org/healthy-lifestyle/nutrition-and-healthy-eating/in-depth/restaurant-dining/art-20044679)

4. Harvard T.H. Chan School of Public Health. "Eating Out: How to Make Healthy Choices."

6.4 Healthy Cooking Techniques: Grilling, Steaming, Roasting, and More

"Healthy cooking is not about sacrificing flavor; it's about enhancing it with fresh, wholesome ingredients and mindful cooking techniques." - Unknown

Introduction:

Healthy cooking techniques play a crucial role in preparing nutritious and flavorful meals while minimizing the use of unhealthy fats and excessive calories. By utilizing cooking methods such as grilling, steaming, roasting, and others, individuals can enhance the taste and texture of foods while preserving their natural flavors and nutrients. Understanding the benefits of various cooking techniques empowers individuals to make healthier choices in the kitchen and promote overall well-being. Exploring healthy cooking techniques provides valuable insights into optimizing meal preparation for delicious and nutritious results.

Key Insights:

1. Grilling: Grilling is a popular cooking method that imparts a smoky flavor to foods without the need for added fats or oils. By grilling lean proteins such as chicken, fish, or vegetables, individuals can create delicious and healthy meals that are low in saturated fats and calories. To further enhance flavor, marinate foods before grilling or season them with herbs, spices, and citrus zest.

2. Steaming: Steaming is a gentle cooking method that preserves the natural flavors, colors, and nutrients of foods while minimizing the use of added fats. Steamed vegetables retain their crisp texture and vibrant appearance, making them an excellent addition to any meal. Steaming is also ideal for cooking delicate proteins such as fish or shellfish, ensuring tender and moist results without the need for excessive oils or sauces.

3. Roasting: Roasting involves cooking foods in the oven at high temperatures, allowing them to caramelize and develop rich flavors. Roasting vegetables enhances their natural sweetness and creates delicious caramelized edges, while roasting meats produces tender and juicy results. To keep roasted dishes healthy, use minimal oil or opt for heart-healthy fats like olive oil, and season with herbs, spices, and aromatics.

4. Sauteing and Stir-Frying: Sauteing and stir-frying involve cooking foods quickly over high heat in a small amount of oil.

These techniques are ideal for cooking vegetables, proteins, and grains, as they retain their texture and nutrients while developing complex flavors. To keep sauteed and stir-fried dishes healthy, use heart-healthy oils such as olive or avocado oil, and incorporate plenty of colorful vegetables and lean proteins.

Conclusion:

Healthy cooking techniques are essential for preparing delicious and nutritious meals that support overall health and well-being. By incorporating methods such as grilling, steaming, roasting, and sauteing into meal preparation, individuals can enhance the taste, texture, and nutritional value of foods while minimizing the use of unhealthy fats and excessive calories. Experimenting with different cooking techniques allows for creativity in the kitchen and opens up a world of flavorful and healthy possibilities for meals that nourish the body and delight the senses.

Resources:

1. American Heart Association. "Healthy Cooking Techniques." (https://www.heart.org/en/healthy-living/healthy-eating/eat-smart/cooking-techniques)

2. Mayo Clinic. "Cooking Techniques for Healthy Eating." (https://www.mayoclinic.org/healthy-lifestyle/nutrition-and-healthy-eating/in-depth/healthy-cooking/art-20049346)

3. EatingWell. "Cooking Techniques for Healthy Eating." (https://www.eatingwell.com/article/288683/cooking-techniques-for-healthy-eating/)

4. Food Network. "Healthy Cooking Techniques."

6.5 Building Balanced Meals: Sample Meal Ideas and Recipes

"Take care of your body. It's the only place you have to live." - Jim Rohn

Introduction:

Building balanced meals is essential for providing the body with the nutrients it needs for optimal health and energy levels throughout the day. Balanced meals incorporate a variety of food groups, including lean proteins, whole grains, healthy fats, and plenty of fruits and vegetables. By combining these components in appropriate portions, individuals can create satisfying and nourishing meals that support overall well-being. Exploring sample meal ideas and recipes offers inspiration and guidance for creating delicious and balanced meals that promote health and vitality.

Key Insights:

1. Protein: Include a source of lean protein in each meal to support muscle repair and satiety. Options include grilled chicken breast, baked fish, tofu, tempeh, beans, lentils, or eggs. Aim to fill one-quarter of your plate with protein-rich foods.

2. Whole Grains: Choose whole grains as the foundation of your meals to provide fiber, vitamins, and minerals. Examples include brown rice, quinoa, whole wheat pasta, barley, bulgur, or farro. Fill another quarter of your plate with whole grains to support sustained energy levels.

3. Vegetables: Load up on colorful vegetables to add flavor, texture, and nutrients to your meals. Aim to fill half of your plate with non-starchy vegetables such as leafy greens, broccoli, bell peppers, carrots, tomatoes, or cucumbers. Experiment with different cooking methods, such as roasting, steaming, or sauteing, to enhance the taste of vegetables.

4. Healthy Fats: Incorporate sources of healthy fats into your meals to support heart health and brain function. Add avocado slices, nuts, seeds, or olive oil to salads, soups, or stir-fries. Use moderation when adding fats to meals, as they are calorie-dense.

Sample Meal Ideas:

1. Grilled Chicken Salad: Grilled chicken breast served over a bed of mixed greens with cherry tomatoes, cucumber slices, avocado, and a drizzle of balsamic vinaigrette.

2. Quinoa Buddha Bowl: Cooked quinoa topped with roasted sweet potatoes, sauteed kale, chickpeas, sliced avocado, and a sprinkle of sesame seeds. Drizzle with tahini dressing for extra flavor.

3. Vegetable Stir-Fry: Stir-fried tofu or tempeh with bell peppers, broccoli, snap peas, carrots, and mushrooms, served over brown rice or quinoa. Season with ginger, garlic, and soy sauce for a flavorful finish.

4. Salmon and Asparagus: Baked salmon fillets with a side of roasted asparagus and quinoa pilaf. Garnish with lemon wedges and fresh herbs for a burst of flavor.

Conclusion:

Building balanced meals is key to supporting overall health and well-being by providing essential nutrients and energy for the body. By incorporating lean proteins, whole grains, plenty of vegetables, and healthy fats into meals, individuals can create satisfying and nourishing dishes that promote vitality and longevity. Experimenting with different meal combinations and recipes allows for creativity in the kitchen and ensures a varied and delicious diet that meets nutritional needs.

Resources:

1. EatingWell. "Quick and Healthy Dinner Recipes." (https://www.eatingwell.com/recipes/17975/cooking-methods -styles/quick-easy/dinner/)

2. Cooking Light. "Healthy Meal Ideas and Recipes." (https://www.cookinglight.com/food/quick-healthy)

3. Food Network. "Healthy Weeknight Meals." (https://www.foodnetwork.com/recipes/photos/healthy-week night-meals)

4. BBC Good Food. "Healthy Meal Ideas." (https://www.bbcgoodfood.com/recipes/collection/healthy-m eal-ideas)

May I Ask You For A Small Favor?

I want to express my sincere gratitude for choosing to invest your time in reading this book. Your decision to explore this work among countless others means a lot to me.

I hope that within these pages, you've discovered actionable insights that can enhance your daily life. Your journey doesn't have to end here, though.

May I kindly request an additional 30 seconds of your valuable time?

Sharing your thoughts about the book through a review would be immensely appreciated. Your review serves as a beacon, guiding other readers to take a chance on my books. It's a small gesture that carries significant weight in the world of authors.

To submit your review effortlessly, please click on the link below. It will take you directly to the book's review page:

"Nutrition for a Vibrant Life"

Alternatively, you can also find the "**Reviews Section**" of this book's page on Amazon.

Your review will require just a minute of your time but will make a monumental difference in helping me connect with a broader audience and I eagerly look forward to reading your review.

Once again, thank you for your unwavering support of my work.

Disclaimer

This book is for educational purposes only. Readers acknowledge that the author does not render legal, financial, medical, or professional advice. The content within this book has been derived from various sources. Please consult a licensed professional before attempting any techniques outlined in this book.

By reading this document, the reader agrees that under no circumstances is the author responsible for any direct or indirect losses incurred as a result of the use of the information contained within this document, including but not limited to errors, omissions, or inaccuracies.

Adherence to all applicable laws and regulations, including international, federal, state, and local governing professional licensing, business practices, advertising, and all other jurisdictions, is the sole responsibility of the purchaser or reader.

Neither the author nor the publisher assumes any responsibility or liability whatsoever on behalf of the purchaser or reader of these materials. Any perceived slight of any individual or organization is purely unintentional.

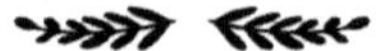